7 Day Detox Miracle: Lose 7 Pounds in 7 Days Safely

Purifying Your Body with the Miracle of Detox

I0427908

Disclaimer

Summary

People become very flustered when they gain weight and don't know how to lose it. It becomes a battle between them and their burgeoning bellies. They start looking for ways to lose weight, but whatever they find doesn't help them. The problems (and their bellies) just keep growing. Then comes a day when they just give up and accept the situation. Now available is a diet that helps you face the situation and not run from it. It's called the 7 Day Detox Miracle Diet to lose 7 pounds eating and drinking healthy meals, teas and shakes. This e-book elaborates on the following subjects:

- Helps you figure out if you need to use the plan or not

- Explains on how you can spot the signs of toxic build up in your body

- Elaborates on the 7 Day Detox Miracle Diet

- Discusses the toxins found in food and drinks and how they get into your body

- Prepares you for the diet by giving you a comprehensive list of the types of things you should purchase from the grocery store during the 7 Day Detox Miracle Diet

- Explains the type of food and drinks you should avid consuming during the 7 Day Detox Miracle Diet

- Provides you with a 7 day meal plan, the specific times you should eat and at what time you should eat

This detox diet provides with healthy meals, tea and shakes that will cleanse your body from within and help you shed 7 pounds. Therefore, if an event is coming up and you want to look your best in just a few days, this diet is for you.

Contents

Introduction to the Detox

Have you started feeling out of sorts lately? As you look in the mirror, you spot various irregularities in yourself such as bloated stomach, blemishes on your skin, constant back pain and other changes in yourself that weren't there before. What on earth could be wrong with you? The answer to your question is fairly simple: your body's toxic removal system is clogged up with waste.

Waste from the air, waste from what you put into your mouth, waste from the lack of exercise and even your genes have made your toxic removal system stop functioning. Your body's toxic prevention system has raised the white flag and the unhealthy eating and exercise patterns have won. Now your body is overloaded with harmful toxins, which it can't get rid of anymore.

The metabolism, which aids in the toxic elimination process, has slowed down, leading to waste accumulation. The body's toxicity-ridding function needs a boost. The boost will help in revitalizing the body and eliminating toxin buildup from it. However, restarting your internal system into functioning correctly may sound like an impossible feat. It may require months or maybe years to clean up the body, since by now the toxic buildup is probably very extensive. What if there was a way to detoxify your body in just 7 days?

In 7 days, you can cleanse your body of the toxins that inhabit it. What's more is that during those 7 days, you can even lose 7 pounds. Therefore, not only will your internal system become clean, but your outer appearance will be changing as well.

The toxins in your body will decrease and so will your weight. All of that in just 7 days if you follow the 7 Day Detox Miracle Diet program where you will eat healthy and look smart doing it. Unlike other diets, this 7 Day Detox Miracle Diet is your best opportunity to cleanse your body of toxins in a safe manner by eating healthy meals.

Do You Need the 7 Day Detox Plan?

When a person's body is going through some unnatural changes where they are feeling more tired and lethargic than usual, they are quick to point the finger at stress for being the culprit. Although it's true stress does cause changes to one's body, stress, however, is not the only culprit.

When people live hectic lives, stress comes as part of the deal. When people are stressed and consumed in their life, they start to adopt unhealthy lifestyles such as eating out, exercising less, watching TV more and going to sleep with a full stomach. Thus, increasing the work of the body's waste elimination system and eventually bringing the system to a steady halt. That's when the body starts sending you "SOS" signals. It wants to bring to your attention that there is something wrong with them and you need to help them.

You might attribute the signals to stress and ignore them. In actuality, those signals are related to the high levels of toxicity and waste present in your system that is unable to get out. Therefore, it's pertinent that you immediately start cleansing your body if you suspect that your body is giving you signals to help them out by releasing the toxins from the body.

High Levels of Toxicity

Following is a list of signals that your body might be giving you:

1. Hemorrhoids

2. Sinus congestion

3. Constipation, bloating and ingestion

4. Headaches and migraines

5. Muscle aches and fatigue

6. Eating too much seafood like tuna or swordfish

7. Dental fillings with mercury

8. Developing food allergies

9. Quick Weight Gain

10. Hormonal imbalances

11. Excess use of Nonsteroidal anti-inflammatory drugs such as ibuprofen

12. Developing skin diseases such as eczema, acne or rosacea

13. Sleepy, lack of energy and extremely tired

14. Loss of focus at work or school

15. Insomnia

16. Fowl breath and strong body odor

17. Weak immune system

18. Depression, stress and anxiety

19. Regular mood swings and crankiness

20. Back and joint pain

If you have any of the illnesses mentioned above, then keep reading to find out how you can decrease the toxicity levels in your body, lose 7 pounds, and become healthy in just 7 days.

Planning Your Detox Diet

When people hear the word "diet," they tend to duck away and hide. Dieting is a difficult and daunting task for many, but without proper nutrition and exercise, the body starts to function backwards. The body can no longer take the burden of junk food, oily food, cold drinks and other poor habits you put it through on a daily basis. Its only defense against your unhealthy eating patterns is to become idle, furthermore giving you an indication that it's time to go into planning mode.

You need to start planning a 7 Day Detox Miracle Diet to help you cleanse your body of wastes and lose up to 7 pounds doing so. Therefore, get on the measuring scale to figure out your body mass index (BMI), learn what you need to buy and what you need to skip at a grocery store and finally set yourself on a weight loss and detoxification journey with delicious appetizing meals and shakes at your side—you won't even feel like you are dieting.

Toxins: The Evil inside Your Body

The presence of toxins in a person's body is the main trigger of hormonal imbalance. An imbalance of the hormonal system changes the way hormones function in the body. Toxins are found in food and the environment.

People's regular interactions with the two leads to rapid weight gain. A weight gain that sometimes people can't even explain why it's happening, as their food consumption compared to others is quite less. Consequently, making it difficult to pinpoint to a specific reason that's causing them to put on weight.

The reason to rapid weight gain lies within them. The toxins have taken over their bodies and have affected their hormones such as testosterone, insulin, thyroid, estrogen and cortisol. Hence, when one hormone fails, the other hormones fail too, as they all function collectively. Following are the names of toxins found in the food or air that can gain access to your body, disrupt the hormonal system and promote weight gain:

1. Phthalates

You can find this ingredient listed on the labels of candles, air fresheners, beauty products and in household cleaners like detergent. These toxins attack the male and female's testosterone levels by decreasing it. This decreases the muscle mass and increases weight.

2. Bisphenol A or BPA

The canned food that people enjoy eating can be quite harmful to a person's internal system. This chemical is not found in the food, but it's found in the lining of the food's container. The chemical uses the food as a means to travel inside your body. Once it's inside your body, it increases the estrogen and insulin levels. In return, your body will begin to develop a resistance to insulin, which means that your body won't be able to control your blood sugar correctly.

3. Pesticides

Farmers spray this chemical on crops to keep the insects from infesting them. This chemical finds its way into people's food and drinks. When people consume the food and drinks, they risk the chance of becoming obese.

4. Artificial Sweeteners

Artificial sweeteners were introduced as form of dietary sugar for people with diabetes or for people who wanted to lose weight. As time passed, the dangers of this synthetic sugar became known. This sugar is found in diet drinks and in diet food. Too much consumption of food and drinks containing this sugar can to lead weight gain.

5. High Fructose Corn Syrup

Intake of high fructose corn syrup can negatively affect a person's liver. When this is consumed on a daily basis, the liver develops a craving for sugar. In addition, a person's metabolism also slows down and the person ends up gaining unwanted weight.

6. Hydrogenated Oils

Hydrogenated oils are better known as Trans fats. These fats are the most dangerous fat-building fats, as they can destroy your metabolism and increase cholesterol levels.

7. Carbohydrates and Refined Sugars

These are the major contributors to rapid weight gain. Food and drinks containing refined sugar and carbs have no nutritional value. In fact, carbs and refined sugars are consumed the most by a majority of people, as they are actively found in junk food, which makes people obese and overweight.

When these toxins exist in your body, the body stops functioning as it used to. Just as you cleanse your face with water to get rid of the sweat, you need to cleanse your body of toxins by using this 7 day miracle plan to lose 7 pounds.

Shop Healthy to Succeed

Before beginning this miracle detox diet, you need to stock up on your food supplies. The first step to starting any diet is making a proper grocery list with items you know will have a profound and changing effect on your body. After only a few days of starting this diet, you will notice a change in your body. In order for this diet to work in your favor, you need to add the following list of food to your diet:

Protein Aisle

1. **Cold-water fish**

2. **Lamb**

3. **Duck**

4. **Turkey**

5. **Organic Poultry**

Dairy Aisle

1. **Coconut Milk**

2. **Almond Milk**

Nuts and Seeds Aisle

1. **Sunflower Seeds**

2. **Sesame Seeds**

3. **Chia Seeds**

4. **Hazelnut**

5. **Pecans**

6. **Almonds**

7. **Cashews**

Gluten-Free Grains Aisle

1. **Brown rice**

2. **Millet**

3. **Tapioca**

4. **Buckwheat**

5. **Potato Flour**

6. **Quinoa**

7. **Oats without Gluten**

Condiments Aisle

1. **Salt**

2. **Pepper**

3. **Vinegar**

4. **Cumin**

5. **Oregano**

6. **Mustard**

7. **Thyme**

8. **Parsley**

9. **Turmeric**

10. **Rosemary**

11. **Basil**

12. **Dill**

13. **Garlic**

14. **Cinnamon**

15. **Tarragon**

16. **Ginger**

Oil Aisle

1. **Olive**

2. **Coconut**

3. **Cod**

4. **Flax**

5. **Safflower**

6. **Sesame**

7. **Almond**

8. **Sunflower**

9. **Walnut**

10. **Canola**

11. **Pumpkin**

Non-Starchy Vegetable Aisle

(Contain fewer calories.)

1. **Zucchini**

2. **Spinach**

3. **Radishes**

4. **Parsley**

5. **Onions**

6. **Mushrooms**

7. **Lettuce**

8. **Kale**

9. **Jalapeno peppers**

10. **Green beans**

11. **Garlic**

12. **Eggplant**

13. **Dandelion greens**

14. **Cucumber**

15. **Celery**

16. **Cauliflower**

17. **Cabbage**

18. **Brussels sprouts**

19. **Broccoli**

20. **Beet greens**

21. **Asparagus**

22. **Arugula**

Starchy Vegetable Aisle

(High in carbohydrates and fiber, but healthy compared to other high-starchy vegetables.)

1. **Lima, Pinto, Black, and Adzuki Beans**

2. **Winter, Acorn, and Acorn Squash**

3. **Turnip**

4. **Carrots**

5. **Chick Peas**

6. **Leeks**

7. **Sweet Potato**

Fruit Aisle

(Choose fruits that are low and moderate in the glycemic index [GI] because they make people feel fuller for longer periods.)

1. **Gooseberries**

2. **Strawberries**

3. **Blueberries**

4. **Raspberries**

5. **Cherries**

6. **Apricots**

7. **Apples**

8. **Melons**

9. **Kiwi Fruit**

10. **Limes**

11. **Lemons**

12. **Pear**

13. **Orange**

Use this list of food items as a guide to help you pick out the correct food when going to the grocery store.

Food's to Avoid Buying During the duration of this detox diet, you should avoid adding these food and drinks into your diet:

1. Do not eat anything containing high-fructose corn syrup.

2. Do not consume any food or drinks that contain artificial sweeteners.

3. Although eating natural sweeteners is okay, however, it's best to avoid them during this detox plan.

4. Avoid drinking caffeinated drinks such as coffee, tea and cola drinks. On the other hand, drinking green tea is allowed because its properties aid the cleansing process.

5. Cut down on all alcohol consumption.

6. Avoid eating food that contains gluten.

7. Do not purchase products that contain flour.

8. Keep junk food as far away from yourself as you can.

9. Do not consume any laxatives or weight loss pills.

10. Do not eat eggs until the detox is over.

11. During the detox diet, do not purchase products containing yeast.

12. Do not purchase dairy products such as butter, cheese, milk and yogurt.

13. Avoid using mayonnaise and butter.

14. Do not purchase peanuts.

For 7 days, which is not a lot, avoiding these food and drinks will thoroughly cleanse your body. Thus, making you feel healthier than ever before. After the diet, if you lower the consumption of these foods, it will promote more weight loss and the chances of toxin build-up in the body will lower.

Beginning Your Detox Miracle Program

The start of anything new can be difficult at first but, with time, it becomes easier. People feel the exact same way about dieting. Moreover, when detoxifying your body, you will be taking away all the food that your body is normally used to eating. You will be consuming smaller meals several times in one day. Here is an idea of how the diet will work:

1. In the morning, you will drink a glass of water.

2. For breakfast, you will drink a shake.

3. For the morning snack, you eat some fresh fruits and drink herbal tea.

4. After an hour, you will drink water again.

5. For lunch, you will eat a light, yet filling salad.

6. For the mid-afternoon snack, you will again drink a glass of water.

7. Before dinner, you drink herbal tea and eat nuts.

8. For dinner, you can eat protein, salad or fish and you will wash down the meal with a glass of purified water.

9. Before going off to bed, you drink herbal tea.

This detox miracle program requires you to eat at specific times in the day. You will be eating something new each day and you will look forward to creating these healthy meals, as they are easy to make.

Day 1: Meal Plan

I.   Morning Water: 7:00 AM

<u>Cinnamon and Apple Water</u>

COOKING TIME

3 minutes

INGREDIENTS

Sliced Apple, 1

Cinnamon Powder, 1/2 tsp

One Large Jug of Purified Water

Ice Cubes

PREPARATION METHOD

1. Slice the apple into 4 parts.

2. Put the sliced apple and the stick of cinnamon in the jar.

3. Cover the sliced apple and the cinnamon powder with ice.

4. Pour purified water into a large jug.

5. Put it in the fridge to drink it chilled.

NUTRITIONAL VALUE PER SERVING

Calories: 98

Fat: 0.0g

Carbohydrates: 26.1g

Protein: 0.1g

II.   Morning Shake: 8:00 AM

Beet Shake

COOKING TIME

6 minutes

INGREDIENTS

Medium Sized Beets, 2

Ginger, 1 inch

Peeled Lemon, 1

Spring of Cilantro Leaves, 1

Ice Cubes

PREPARATION METHOD

1. Put all of the ingredients in the blender and grind them all together.

NUTRITIONAL VALUE PER SERVING

Calories: 98

Fat: 0.0g

Carbohydrates: 21.8g

Protein: 4.2g

III. Morning Snack and Drink: 10:00 AM

a) **Ginger and Lemon Herbal Tea**

COOKING TIME

10 minutes

INGREDIENTS

Boiling Water, 4 cups

Lemon Juice, 3 tbsp

Ginger (grated,) 4 tbsp

Lemon and Lime Slices, (garnishing)

PREPARATION METHOD

1. Pour the water in a pot and put it on the stove to boil.

2. Pour the lemon juice and grated ginger in it.

3. Let the water boil for a few minutes.

4. Use the sieve to pour in the herbal tea into the cup.

5. Use the slices of lemon and lime as garnish and put it on the sides of the cup or directly in the cup.

6. You can drink this tea either chilled or hot.

NUTRITIONAL VALUE PER SERVING

Calories: 86

Fat: 1.7g

Carbohydrates: 16.2g

Protein: 2.3g

b) **Raspberries**

INGREDIENTS

Raspberries, 1 cup

NUTRITIONAL VALUE PER SERVING

Calories: 52

Fat: 0.7g

Carbohydrates: 12.0g

Protein: 1.0g

*At 11:00 AM, drink the cinnamon and apple water.

Lunch: 12:00 PM

Refreshing Cherry and Cucumber Salad

COOKING TIME

20 minutes

INGREDIENTS

Diced Cucumber, 1

Medium Sliced Red Onions, 4 tbsp

Mint Leaves, chopped 1 tbsp

Halved Cherry Tomatoes, 2-3

Sliced Tomato, 1

PREPARATION METHOD

1. Take the cucumber, peel and slice it.

2. Put the cucumber, tomato and red onions in the bowl.

3. Take the mint leaves and put them in the bowl.

4. Put them in the fridge to cool the salad.

NUTRITIONAL VALUE PER SERVING

Calories: 132

Fat: 1.7g

Carbohydrates: 29.6g

Protein: 5.9g

*At 2:00 PM, drink the beet shake again.

*At 4:00 PM, drink the ginger and lemon herbal tea that you drank in the morning and eat 15 cashews.

Dinner: 6:00 PM

Ginger Carrot Soup

COOKING TIME

20 minutes

INGREDIENTS

Olive Oil, 1 tbsp

Cloves of garlic, 4

Onion (chopped), 1

Water, 4 cups

Salt, 1/2 tsp

Carrots, 2

Garbanzo beans, 2 lbs

Agave nectar, 1 tbsp

PREPARATION METHOD

1. Spread the olive oil in a large pot.
2. Chop and peel the ginger and garlic.
3. Chop the onion.
4. Peel the carrots and chop them into big chunks.
5. Now, add the onion, ginger and garlic into the pot.
6. After 5 minutes when the onion turn a little red, add the carrots.
7. Next, add all the other ingredients and wait for the carrots to soften.

8. Mix the soup well and serve with a cold glass of water.

NUTRITIONAL VALUE PER SERVING

Calories: 141

Fat: 3.5g

Carbohydrates: 23.5g

Protein: 5g

*At 8:00 PM, before going to bed, drink the ginger and herbal tea again.

Day 2: Meal Plan

I. Morning Drink: 7:00 AM

Berry Lime Water

COOKING TIME

3 minutes

INGREDIENTS

Water, 2 1/2 cup

Strawberries, 1 1/2 cup

Mint leaves, 3 cups

Ice Cubes

PREPARATION METHOD

1. Halve the strawberries and put them into a jug.

2. Put the water into the jug and fill it up with water.

3. Put it in the fridge to drink it chilled.

NUTRITIONAL VALUE PER SERVING

Calories: 79

Fat: 0.8g

Carbohydrates: 18.4g

Protein: 2.2g

II. Morning Shake: 8:00 AM

Hawaiian Shake

COOKING TIME

6 minutes

INGREDIENTS

Banana, 1 cup

Pineapple pieces, 1 cup

Mango Chunks, 13 pieces

Organic green grapes, 1/2 cup

Concentrated Orange Juice, 2 tbsp

Organic Kale, 1 cup

Almond Milk (unsweetened), 2 cups

PREPARATION METHOD

1. Put all of the ingredients in the blender and grind them all together.

NUTRITIONAL VALUE PER SERVING

Calories: 113

Fat: 2g

Carbohydrates: 4g

Protein: 3g

III. Morning Snack and Drink: 10:00 AM

a) Fresh Mint Ginger and Fennel Herbal Tea

COOKING TIME

10 minutes

INGREDIENTS

Boiling Water, 1 cup

Mint Leaf, 2 tsp

Fennel Seeds, 1/2 tsp

Dried Ginger, 1/2 tsp

PREPARATION METHOD

1. Pour the water in a pot and put it on the stove to boil.

2. Put the fennel seeds, dried ginger and mint leaves in a cup.

3. Turn off the stove and pour the boiling water into the cup.

4. With a plate or a lid cover the cup for 6 minutes.

5. Take the lid off and enjoy your herbal tea.

NUTRITIONAL VALUE PER SERVING

Calories: 8

Fat: 0.2g

Carbohydrates: 1.5g

Protein: 0.4g

b) **Strawberries**

INGREDIENTS

Strawberries 1 cup

NUTRITIONAL VALUE PER SERVING

Calories: 46

Fat: 0.4g

Carbohydrates: 11.1g

Protein: 1.0g

*At 11:00 AM, drink the berry lime water.

IV.   Lunch: 12:00 PM

<u>Colorful Salad</u>

COOKING TIME

15 minutes

INGREDIENTS

Cabbage, 1 cup

Chopped Romaine, 1 cup

Diced Red Bell Pepper (medium), 1/4 cup

Avocado, 1/2 cup

Sesame Seeds, 1 tsp

PREPARATION METHOD

1. In a bowl, place the shredded cabbage.

2. Next put the chopped romaine and diced red bell pepper in the bowl.

3. Cut the avocado in half and put it on top of the other ingredients in the bowl.

4. Now put the sesame seeds in the bowl.

5. Then salt and pepper to taste.

NUTRITIONAL VALUE PER SERVING

Calories: 175

Fat: 15.9g

Carbohydrates: 8.8g

Protein: 2.6g

*At 2:00 PM, drink the Hawaiian shake.

*At 4:00 PM, drink the fresh mint ginger and fennel herbal tea and eat 15 hazelnuts.

V.   Dinner: 6:00 PM

Mexican Corn Tortilla

COOKING TIME

20 minutes

INGREDIENTS

Hummus, 2 tbsp

Tortillas (corn), 4

Beans, 2 tbsp

Cilantro (chopped), 2 tbsp

Spinach, 2 tbsp

Salsa, 4 tsp

PREPARATION METHOD

1. With a knife, spread hummus on the first tortilla.

2. Now, put the beans on the second tortilla.

3. Do the same with the two remaining tortillas.

4. On the tortilla with the hummus, put the salsa, cilantro and spinach on it.

5. Cook each tortilla on a skillet for about 2 minutes on medium heat.

NUTRITIONAL VALUE PER SERVING

Calories: 172

Fat: 0.5g

Carbohydrates: 31g

Protein: 6g

*At 8:00 PM, before going to bed, drink the fresh mint ginger and fennel herbal tea again.

Day 3: Meal Plan

I. Morning Drink: 7:00 AM

Minty Lemony Cucumber Water

COOKING TIME

5 minutes

INGREDIENTS

Water, 12 cups

Sliced Lemons, 3

Sliced Cucumber (small), 1

Mint Leaves, 12

PREPARATION METHOD

1. Take the lemons and cucumbers and wash them well before slicing them.

2. Put the slices of lemon, cucumber and the mint leaves into the jug.

3. Fill the jug with water and ice and put it in the fridge to cool the drink.

NUTRITIONAL VALUE PER SERVING

Calories: 52

Protein: 2.0g

Carbohydrates: 13.0g

Fat: 0.6g

II. Morning Shake: 8:00 AM

Citrus Cucumber Shake

COOKING TIME

6 minutes

INGREDIENTS

Carrots, 3

Cucumber, 1/2 cup

Orange, 2

Ginger, 1/2 piece

Cold Water, 1 cup

Ice Cubes

PREPARATION METHOD

1. Don't unpeel the carrots, instead scrub them with water and cut them into big chunks.

2. Cut the unpeeled cucumber in half.

3. Peel the oranges and ginger.

4. Put all the ingredients in the blender.

5. Put the water in the blender with some ice cubes.

6. Blend everything together and drink up.

NUTRITIONAL VALUE PER SERVING

Calories: 169g

Protein: 3.8g

Carbohydrates: 41.1g

Fat: 0.8g

III.   Morning Snack and Drink: 10:00 AM

a) **Flowered Chamomile Herbal Tea**

COOKING TIME

10 minutes

INGREDIENTS

Chamomile Flowers, 1 tbsp

Hot Water, 1 cup

Small Apple, sliced 1

PREPARATION METHOD

1. Wash the flowers with purified water.

2. In the teapot, boil the water.

3. Put the slices of apple in a bowl and smash them.

4. Put the smashed apple into the boiling water.

5. Cover the teapot and let the water boil for 3 minutes.

6. Pour the tea into cups.

NUTRITIONAL VALUE PER SERVING

Calories: 78

Fat: 0.2g

Carbohydrates: 20.6g

Protein: 0.0g

b) **Lettuce**

INGREDIENTS

Lettuce, lightly fried, 1 cup

Olive Oil, 1 tsp

NUTRITIONAL VALUE PER SERVING

Calories: 48

Fat: 4.8g

Carbohydrates: 1.6g

Protein: 0.5g

*At 11:00 AM, drink minty lemony cucumber water.

IV.   Lunch: 12:00 PM

Green, White, and Red Salad

COOKING TIME

20 minutes

INGREDIENTS

Broccoli, 1/4 cup

Cauliflower, 1/2 cup

Shredded Carrots, 1/4 cup

Currants, 1/2 cup

Parsley, 1/4 cup

Lemon Juice, 1 tbsp

PREPARATION METHOD

1. Take the stems off the broccoli and cauliflower, chop them and put them in a bowl.

2. Shred the carrots using a shredder and put them in the bowl.

3. Mix in the parsley, lemon juice and currants.

NUTRITIONAL VALUE PER SERVING

Calories: 145

Fat: 1.1g

Carbohydrates: 30.3g

Protein: 9.3g

*At 2:00 PM, drink the citrus cucumber shake.

*At 4:00 PM, drink the flowered chamomile tea herbal tea and eat 15 sunflower seeds.

V.   Dinner: 6:00 PM

Beet Soup

COOKING TIME

20 minutes

INGREDIENTS

Medium Beets, 1

Diced Small Shallot, 1/2 cup

Chopped Garlic Clove, 1 tsp

Apple Cider, 1 tsp

Salt, 1 tsp

Parsley, 2 tbsp

Coconut Milk, 1/4 cup

PREPARATION METHOD

1. Take the beets, peel them and cut them into four parts.

2. In a pot, put some water to heat (about an inch).

3. Put the shallots, garlic and beet in the boiling water.

4. Close the lid to steam the vegetables.

5. Put the steamed vegetables in a blender with some water.

6. Dump in the parsley and vinegar into the blender and blend on high speed.

7. While blending, remember to keep adding coconut milk.

8. After its ready, put it in a bowl and quench your thirst with a large glass of purified water.

NUTRITIONAL VALUE PER SERVING

Calories: 147

Fat: 14.4g

Carbohydrates: 5.4g

Protein: 1.8g

*At 8:00 PM, before going to bed, drink the flowery chamomile herbal tea.

Day 4: Meal Plan

I. Morning Drink: 7:00 AM

Straw-Melon-Berry Water

COOKING TIME

5 minutes

INGREDIENTS

Strawberries, 1/2 cup

Watermelon, 2 cups

Rosemary, 2 tbsp

Water, 2 cups

PREPARATION METHOD

1. Mix the strawberries and rosemary in a bowl.

2. Put the watermelon in the jug.

3. Put the strawberries and rosemary in the jug.

4. Pour in cold water.

5. Put it in the fridge to cool for 15 minutes.

NUTRITIONAL VALUE PER SERVING

Calories: 121

Protein: 2.4g

Carbohydrates: 29.8g

Fat: 1.0g

II. Morning Shake: 8:00 AM

Green Grass Shake

COOKING TIME

6 minutes

INGREDIENTS

Apple, 1

Lemon Juice, 1

Kale, 1 cup

Celery (small), 1

Cilantro, 1/3 cup

Chia Seed, 1 tbsp

Cinnamon (grounded), 1/4 tsp

PREPARATION METHOD

1. Put all of the ingredients in the blender and grind them all together.

NUTRITIONAL VALUE PER SERVING

Calories: 135

Protein: 2.3g

Carbohydrates: 34.0g

Fat: 0.1g

III. Morning Snack and Drink: 10:00 AM

a) **Sour Lemon Herbal Tea**

COOKING TIME

10 minutes

INGREDIENTS

Water, 2 cups

Apple Cider Vinegar, 2 tsp

Packet of tea (organic), 1

Stevia leaves, 1 tsp

Lemon, 1 tbsp

PREPARATION METHOD

1. Mix all of the ingredients in a blender.

2. Drink it either cold or hot.

NUTRITIONAL VALUE PER SERVING

Calories: 13

Fat: 0.0g

Carbohydrates: 4.2g

Protein: 0.3g

b) **Pears**

INGREDIENTS

Pears (halved), 1 cup

NUTRITIONAL VALUE PER SERVING

Calories: 93

Fat: 0.2g

Carbohydrates: 24.9g

Protein: 0.6g

*At 11:00 AM, drink straw-melon-berry water.

Lunch: 12:00 PM

Tofu Salad

COOKING TIME

10 minutes

INGREDIENTS

Grape seed Oil, 2 tsp

Tofu (organic), 1/2 cup

Dill Weed, 1/2 tsp

Spinach, 6 oz

Cabbage, 10 oz

Beets (small), 8 oz

Balsamic Vinegar, 1/4 cup

Walnuts, 1/4 cup

Salt to taste

PREPARATION METHOD

9. In a skillet, pour the grape seed oil.

10. Once the oil heats, put in the dill, salt and tofu into it.

11. When the tofu begins to brown, turn off the stove.

NUTRITIONAL VALUE PER SERVING

Calories: 176

Fat: 9.5g

Carbohydrates: 4.5g

Protein: 9.5g

*At 2:00 PM, drink the green grass shake.

*At 4:00 PM, drink the sour lemon herbal tea and eat 15 almonds.

VI.   Dinner: 6:00 PM

<u>Vegetable Delight</u>

COOKING TIME

20 minutes

INGREDIENTS

Olive Oil, 1 tbsp

Onion (diced), 1

Garlic Cloves (minced), 2

Curry Powder, 2 tbsp

Tomatoes, 2 (chopped)

Carrots, 3 (diced)

Purified Water, 3 cups

Celery, 3 (sliced)

Packed of Mixed Green Veggies, 16 oz

2 packets of Lentils (steamed), 17.6 oz

Salt, 1 tsp

PREPARATION METHOD

1. In a large pot, sauté the minced garlic, curry powder and diced onion in olive oil for 5 minutes.

2. Add the rest of the ingredients into the pot, including the water.

3. Close the lid and let it cook for 12 minutes.

4. Take it out and serve with a large glass of purified water.

NUTRITIONAL VALUE PER SERVING

Calories: 145

Fat: 1.5g

Carbohydrates: 23.5g

Protein: 9.5g

*At 8:00 PM, before going to bed, drink the sour lemon herbal tea.

Day 5: Meal Plan

I.   Morning Drink: 7:00 AM

Minty Vinegar Water

COOKING TIME

5 minutes

INGREDIENTS

Lemon (sliced), 1

Cucumber (sliced), 1/2 cup

Mint Leaf (whole), 4

Apple Cider Vinegar, 3 tbsp

Purified Water, 8 cups

PREPARATION METHOD

1. Take the cucumber and lemon and thinly slice them.

2. Put the sliced cucumber and into the jug.

3. Now, pick up the mint leaves and put them in the jug.

4. Fill the jug up with water.

5. Lastly, put apple cider vinegar into the jar.

6. Pour in cold water.

7. Put it in the fridge to cool for 15 minutes or add ice and drink it right away.

NUTRITIONAL VALUE PER SERVING

Calories: 54

Protein: 0.6g

Carbohydrates: 10.3g

Fat: 0.6g

II.   Morning Shake: 8:00 AM

Green Tea Shake

COOKING TIME

6 minutes

INGREDIENTS

Green tea, 1 cup (2 tea bags)

Ice, 2 cups

Peaches, 2 (unpeeled)

Banana, 1

PREPARATION METHOD

1. Put all of the ingredients in the blender and grind them all together.

NUTRITIONAL VALUE PER SERVING

Calories: 47

Protein: 5.4g

Carbohydrates: 1.6g

Fat: 0g

III.   Morning Snack and Drink: 10:00 AM

a) Lemon Ginger Herbal Tea

COOKING TIME

10 minutes

INGREDIENTS

Coriander Seeds, 2 tsp

Fennel Seeds, 2 tsp

Cumin Seeds (whole), 1/4 tsp

Black Peppercorns, 1 tsp

Water, 1 cup

Lemon (sliced), 1

Ginger (sliced), 3 tbsp

Mint Leaves, 8 tbsp

PREPARATION METHOD

1. Combine all the dry ingredients together in a cup.

2. Put 1 cup of water into a pot on medium-high heat and let it boil.

3. Now take the ginger and the meat leaves to mash them together.

4. Once the water starts boiling, put the dry ingredients and the mint-ginger mash into the pot.

5. Again let the water boil.

6. After a few minutes turn off the stove and cover the pot with a lid for another few minutes.

7. Finally, pour the tea into a cup, put the lemon slices in it and sip

.NUTRITIONAL VALUE PER SERVING

Calories: 53

Fat: 1.3g

Carbohydrates: 13.7g

Protein: 3.2g

a) **Green Apple**

INGREDIENTS

Green Apple (sliced), 1

NUTRITIONAL VALUE PER SERVING

Calories: 95

Fat: 0.0g

Carbohydrates: 25.1g

Protein: 0.0g

*At 11:00 AM, drink the minty vinegar water.

Lunch: 12:00 PM

Bean Salad

COOKING TIME

10 minutes

INGREDIENTS

Purple Onion (diced), 1/2 cup

Red Bell Pepper (diced), 1

Pinto Beans (15-oz), 1

Kidney Beans (15-oz), 1

Green Soy Beans, 1 cup

Low-fat vinaigrette dressing, 1/4 cup

Salt, 1/8 tsp

PREPARATION METHOD

1. In a bowl mix all the ingredients

2. Put it in the fridge to cool

NUTRITIONAL VALUE PER SERVING

Calories: 216

Fat: 3.5g

Carbohydrates: 35.5g

Protein: 13g

*At 2:00 PM, drink the green tea shake.

*At 4:00 PM, drink the lemon ginger herbal tea and eat 15 sesame seeds.

VII.   Dinner: 6:00 PM

<u>Salmon Delight</u>

COOKING TIME

20 minutes

INGREDIENTS

Onions (diced), 1 cup

Tamari Soy Sauce (organic/wheat-free), 1 tsp

Apple Cider Vinegar, 1/2 cup

Cucumbers (sliced), 2

Garlic (minced), 4 cloves

Salmon Fillets, 1 lb

Ginger, 2 tsp

Olive Oil, 1 tsp

PREPARATION METHOD

1. Combine the apple cider vinegar, ginger, garlic and tamari soy sauce into a pan.
2. When the pan starts to boil, quickly stir it and take it off the heat after 3 minutes.
3. Put the cucumbers in the pan.
4. Now, take the salmon and dab it each side of the fish with olive oil. Don't drench it in oil, but lightly with your hand put the oil on the salmon.
5. Broil each side of the salmon for 5 minutes until it's fully cooked.

NUTRITIONAL VALUE PER SERVING

Calories: 139

Fat: 5.6g

Carbohydrates: 6.6g

Protein: 15.5g

*At 8:00 PM, before going to bed, drink the lemon ginger herbal tea.

Day 6: Meal Plan

I.   Morning Drink: 7:00 AM

<u>Tangy Grapefruit Water</u>

COOKING TIME

5 minutes

INGREDIENTS

Water, 24 cups

Grapefruit, 6 wedges

Tangerine, 1 cup

Cucumber (sliced), 1/2 cup

Peppermint leaves, 2 tbsp

PREPARATION METHOD

1. Wash the grapefruit, cucumber, tangerine and mint leaves with purified water.
2. Slice the cucumber and tangerine.
3. Take a jug and put all the ingredients into it.
4. Fill the jug with the water.
5. If able to, let the ingredients soak in the water for at least 2 hours in the fridge.

NUTRITIONAL VALUE PER SERVING

Calories: 53

Protein: 1.1g

Carbohydrates: 13.3g

Fat: 0.2g

II.   Morning Shake: 8:00 AM

Gooseberry Mint Shake

COOKING TIME

6 minutes

INGREDIENTS

Gooseberry (large), 7

Lemon zest, 1/2 tsp

Sliced lemon, 1/2

Cold water, 7 cups

Salt, 1 tbsp

Mint Leaves (sprigs), 2

PREPARATION METHOD

1. Put all of the ingredients in the blender and grind them all together.

NUTRITIONAL VALUE PER SERVING

Calories: 84

Protein: 0.4g

Carbohydrates: 18.8g

Fat: 0.1g

III. Morning Snack and Drink: 10:00 AM

a) **Turmeric Herbal Tea**

COOKING TIME

10 minutes

INGREDIENTS

Ginger root, 2 tsp

Turmeric Powder, 2 tsp

Cayenne Pepper, 1 tsp

Lemon Juice, 3

Sliced lemon, 1

Water, 8 cups

PREPARATION METHOD

1. For this tea, use a juicer to juice ginger root with the three lemons.
2. In a large jug, add the lemon and ginger mixture to the 8 cups of water already in it.
3. Add cayenne pepper and the sliced lemon into the jug.
4. Mix it well and pour it in a cup to drink.

NUTRITIONAL VALUE PER SERVING

Calories: 26

Fat: 0.8g

Carbohydrates: 5.0g

Protein: 0.7g

b) **Melons**

INGREDIENTS

Melon (sliced) 1 cup

NUTRITIONAL VALUE PER SERVING

Calories: 53

Fat: 0.3g

Carbohydrates: 12.7g

Protein: 1.3g

*At 11:00 AM, drink the tangy grapefruit water.

Lunch: 12:00 PM

<u>Lightly Grilled Eggplant</u>

COOKING TIME

10 minutes

INGREDIENTS

Eggplant, 1 large

Cloves of garlic (minced) 2

Olive Oil, 3 tbsp

Salt, 1/4 tsp

Balsamic Vinegar, 3 tbsp

Black Pepper, 1 tsp

PREPARATION METHOD

1. Set the gas stove on high and preheat it.
2. Take the eggplant and cut thick slices.
3. In a medium size bowl, put the olive oil, vinegar, salt, garlic cloves and pepper.
4. Stir all of the ingredients in the bowl together.
5. Take the thick slices you cut and baste it with the mixture.
6. Put it on the gas stove and let it grill for 11-13 minutes.

NUTRITIONAL VALUE PER SERVING

Calories: 82

Fat: 7.2g

Carbohydrates: 4.8g

Protein: 0.8g

*At 2:00 PM, drink the gooseberry mint shake.

*At 4:00 PM, drink the turmeric herbal tea and eat 15 sesame seeds.

VIII.   Dinner: 6:00 PM

<u>Halibut Heaven</u>

COOKING TIME

20 minutes

INGREDIENTS

Cloves of Garlic, 3

Pepper, 1 tsp

Olive Oil, 1 tbsp

Lime Juice, 1/4 cup

Basil Leaves, 1 1/4 cup

Halibut Steaks, 1 1/2 lbs

Salt, 1 tbsp

PREPARATION METHOD

1. In a large dish, put all of the ingredients in it except for the halibut.
2. Now, put the halibut in the dish and leave it in there to marinate it for 2 hours.
3. Next, grill the fish while changing the sides every five minutes to ensure that it's fully cooked.
4. Warm the leftover marinade in a microwave and pour over the fish.

NUTRITIONAL VALUE PER SERVING

Calories: 226

Fat: 6g

Carbohydrates: 35g

Protein: 37g

*At 8:00 PM, before going to bed, drink the turmeric herbal tea.

Day 7: Meal Plan

I.   Morning Drink: 7:00 AM

Kiwi Strawberry Water

COOKING TIME

5 minutes

INGREDIENTS

Water, 8 cups

Strawberries, 2

Kiwis, 2

PREPARATION METHOD

1. Cut strawberries and kiwis in half
2. Put them in a jug
3. Pour the water over the strawberries and kiwis in the jug
4. Either put the jug in the fridge or put some ice into the jug to make it cool.

NUTRITIONAL VALUE PER SERVING

Calories: 13

Protein: 0.2g

Carbohydrates: 3.0g

Fat: 0.1g

II.   Morning Shake: 8:00 AM

Mix Berries Shake

COOKING TIME

6 minutes

INGREDIENTS

Mix berries, 2 cups

Pomegranate Juice (unsweetened), 1 cup

PREPARATION METHOD

1. Put all of the ingredients in the blender and grind them all together.

NUTRITIONAL VALUE PER SERVING

Calories: 75

Protein: 0.0g

Carbohydrates: 18.5g

Fat: 0.0g

III.   Morning Snack and Drink: 10:00 AM

a) <u>Whole Spice Herbal Tea</u>

COOKING TIME

10 minutes

INGREDIENTS

Water, 8 cups

Cumin Seed (whole), 1/4 tsp

Coriander (whole), 1/2 tsp

Fennel Seed (whole), 1/2 tsp

Cardamom pods, 5

PREPARATION METHOD

1. Boil the water and put all the ingredients in it.
2. Let the water continue to boil for a few minutes.
3. Then using a sieve transfer all the tea into the cup.
4. Throw away the used spices and enjoy your tea.

NUTRITIONAL VALUE PER SERVING

Calories: 14

Fat: 0.3g

Carbohydrates: 2.8g

Protein: 0.5g

b) Peaches

INGREDIENTS

Peaches (sliced), 1 cup

NUTRITIONAL VALUE PER SERVING

Calories: 66

Fat: 0.4g

Carbohydrates: 16.2g

Protein: 1.6g

*At 11:00 AM, drink the kiwi strawberry water.

Lunch: 12:00 PM

Cabbage and Avocado Salad

COOKING TIME

10 minutes

INGREDIENTS

Cabbage (shredded), 3 cups

Yellow and Red Peppers, 1/4 cup

Avocado (diced), 1 1/2 cup

Lime Juice, 1

Hemp Seed (organic), 1/4 cup

Cilantro, 3 tbsp

PREPARATION METHOD

1. Take the avocado and mash until it gets a creamy texture.
2. Put all the ingredients in a large bowl except for the avocado cream.
3. Now, pour the avocado cream into the bowl and combine it with everything.

NUTRITIONAL VALUE PER SERVING

Calories: 212

Fat: 18.2g

Carbohydrates: 11g

Protein: 4.7g

*At 2:00 PM, drink the mixed berries shake.

*At 4:00 PM, drink the whole spice herbal tea and eat 15 almonds.

IX.   Dinner: 6:00 PM

Sweet Potato Soup

COOKING TIME

20 minutes

INGREDIENTS

Sweet Potatoes (small), 5

Purified water, 1 cup

Onion, small (chopped), 1

Garlic Cloves, 3

Curry Powder, 2 tsp

Salt, 1/2 tsp

Cilantro (garnishing), 1/4 cup

PREPARATION METHOD

1. Put all of the ingredients except for the cilantro into a large pot.
2. Put the water into the pot and turn on the heat.
3. In the water, let the sweet potatoes boil until they become soft and you are able to put a knife through it easily.
4. Now, transfer everything from the pot into a blender.
5. Again, transfer the soup from the blender to the pot to heat it a little before serving.
6. Drink a large glass of purified water with your meal.

NUTRITIONAL VALUE PER SERVING

Calories: 64

Fat: 0g

Carbohydrates: 14.5g

Protein: 1.5g

*At 8:00 PM, before going to bed, drink the whole spice herbal tea.

Conclusion

The detox diet, if followed correctly, can yield great results in just 7 days. Your mood will brighten and you will notice an increase in energy. You will look and feel radiant. You will actually see and feel the toxins exiting out of your body. The exiting of toxins from one's body is associated with some common symptoms a person gets at the beginning of the detox diet.

The first few days of this diet, you may feel constipated, nauseous, hunger, fatigue, bad breath and even irritability. Be assured that this is completely normal and the symptoms dissipate quickly. To better deal with the symptoms, drink plenty of water. That's why this 7 Day Miracle Detox Diet focuses on drinking herbal tea 3 times a day and a large glass of cold purified water with every meal. You will look and feel 7 pounds lighter in just 7 days.

That's definitely a miracle alright.

*Note: Before starting this detox diet, consult your doctor if you are pregnant, feeding, have an illness, take certain medication or are a young child or older than 65.